The Complete Anti-Inflammatory Vegetarian Recipes Book

50 Quick and Simple Vegetarian Recipes to enjoy your diet in the best way

Natalie Worley

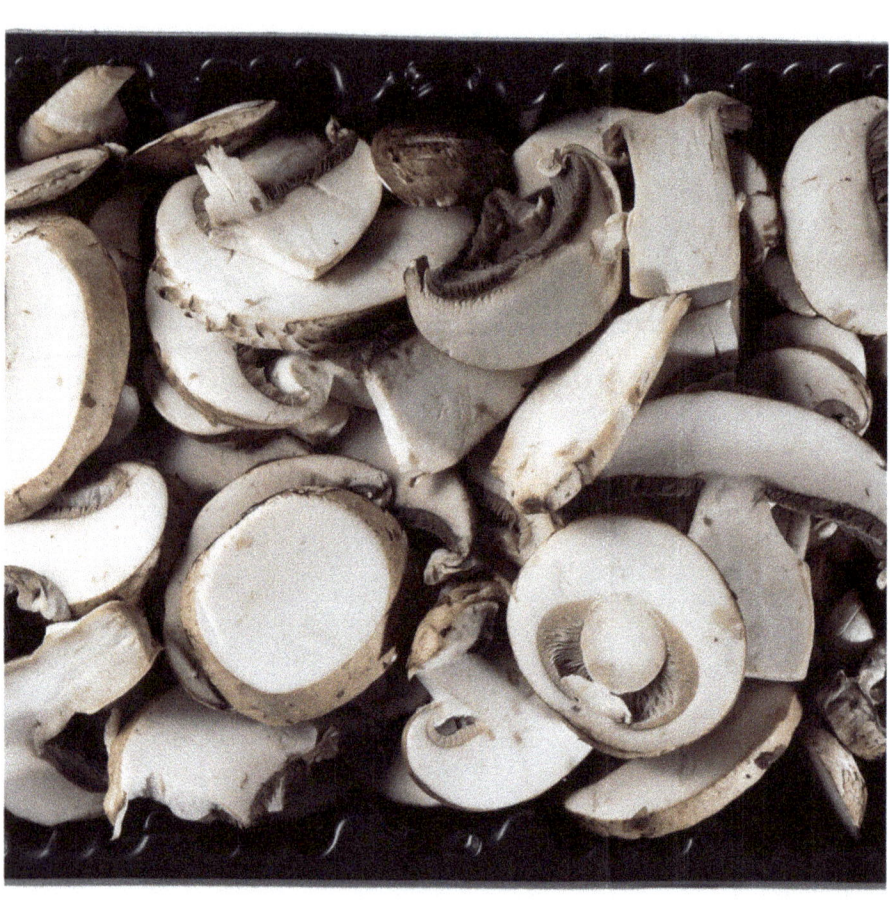

© copyright 2021 – all rights reserved.

the content contained within this book may not be reproduced, duplicated or transmitted without direct written permission from the author or the publisher.

under no circumstances will any blame or legal responsibility be held against the publisher, or author, for any damages, reparation, or monetary loss due to the information contained within this book. either directly or indirectly.

legal notice:

this book is copyright protected. this book is only for personal use. you cannot amend, distribute, sell, use, quote or paraphrase any part, or the content within this book, without the consent of the author or publisher.

disclaimer notice:

please note the information contained within this document is for educational and entertainment purposes only. all effort has been executed to present accurate, up to date, and reliable, complete information. no warranties of any kind are declared or implied. readers acknowledge that the author is not engaging in the rendering of legal, financial, medical or professional advice. the content within this book has been derived from various sources. please consult a licensed professional before attempting any techniques outlined in this book.

by reading this document, the reader agrees that under no circumstances is the author responsible for any losses, direct or indirect, which are incurred as a result of the use of information contained within this document, including, but not limited to, — errors, omissions, or inaccuracies.

Table of Contents

Baked Avocado 6

Baked Cremini Mushrooms 7

Bean Spread 9

Eggplant Balls 11

Spicy Artichoke 14

Mushrooms Cakes 16

Baked Grapes 18

Green Peas Paste 19

Baked Butternut Squash 20

Cauliflower Balls 21

Baked Eggplants 24

Zucchini Cakes 25

Baked Jalapenos 27

Baked Onions 28

Mushroom Steaks 29

Baked Turnip 31

Avocado Spread 32

Burrito Bowl 34

Grilled Peppers 36

Parsley Guacamole 38

Baked Chickpeas 39

Broccoli Steaks 41

Lemon Bok Choy 43

Tomato & Mushroom Soup 45

Broccoli & Cheese Soup 47

Red Lentils with Spinach 49

Vegetarian Balls in Gravy 51

Quinoa with Veggies 56

Quinoa with Asparagus 58

Quinoa & Beans with Veggies 60

- Coconut Brown Rice 62
- Brown Rice & Cherries Pilaf 64
- Brown Rice Casserole 67
- Rice, Lentils & Veggie Casserole 70
- Herbed Bulgur Pilaf 74
- Zoodles 77
- Biryani 79
- Greek Mixed Roasted Vegetables 83
- Autumn Roasted Green Beans 86
- Roasted Summer Squash 88
- Savory Baked Acorn Squash 89
- Roasted Brussels Sprouts 90
- Roasted Rosemary Potatoes 92
- Sweet Potato Wedges 95
- Best Lentil Curry 97
- Chana Masala 99
- Zucchini Noodle Pasta with Avocado Pesto 101
- Thai Soup 103
- Vegan Lasagna 105
- Caprese Zoodles 107

Baked Avocado

Prep Time: 10 min | **Cook Time:** 20 min | **Serve:** 4

- 2 avocados, peeled, pitted, halved
- 1 tablespoon olive oil
- ½ teaspoon dried thyme

1. Put the avocado halves in the baking tray and sprinkle with olive oil and dried thyme.
2. Bake the avocados at 365F for 120 minutes.

Nutrition: 235 calories, 1.9g protein, 8.7g carbohydrates, 23.1g fat, 6.8g fiber, 0mg cholesterol, 6mg sodium, 488mg potassium

Baked Cremini Mushrooms

Prep Time: 10 min | **Cook Time:** 30 min | **Serve:** 4

- 3 cups cremini mushrooms
- ¼ cup plain yogurt
- ¼ cup fresh parsley, chopped
- 1 teaspoon minced garlic
- 1 teaspoon ground turmeric
- 1 tablespoon olive oil

1.Mix cremini mushrooms with plain yogurt, parsley, and all remaining ingredients.

2.Put the mixture in the tray and bake at 350F for 30 minutes.

Nutrition: 60 calories, 2.4g protein, 4.1g carbohydrates, 3.8g fat, 0.6g fiber, 1mg cholesterol, 16mg sodium, 315mg potassium

Bean Spread

Prep Time: 10 min | **Cook Time:** 0 min | **Serve:** 6

- 2 cups red kidney beans, boiled
- 3 tablespoons plain yogurt
- 1 teaspoon ground nutmeg
- 1 teaspoon cayenne pepper
- 1 tablespoon fresh cilantro, chopped

1. Blend the red kidney beans until you get a smooth paste.
2. Then mix the beans with plain yogurt, ground nutmeg, cayenne pepper, and cilantro.
3. Carefully mix the spread.

Nutrition: 215 calories, 14.3g protein, 38.5g carbohydrates, 0.9g fat, 9.5g fiber, 0mg cholesterol, 13mg sodium, 860mg potassium

Eggplant Balls

Prep Time: 10 min | **Cook Time:** 5 min | **Serve:** 6

- 2 cups eggplants, peeled, boiled
- ½ cup almond flour
- 1 teaspoon ground cumin
- ½ teaspoon ground coriander
- 1 teaspoon chili powder
- 1 tablespoon olive oil

1. Blend the eggplant until smooth and mix it with almond flour, ground cumin, ground coriander, and chili powder.
2. Make the small balls.
3. After this, preheat the olive oil in the skillet well.

4.Put the eggplant balls inside and roast them for 2 minutes per side.

Nutrition: 86 calories, 2.4g protein, 4g carbohydrates, 7g fat, 2.2g fiber, 0mg cholesterol, 9mg sodium, 77mg potassium

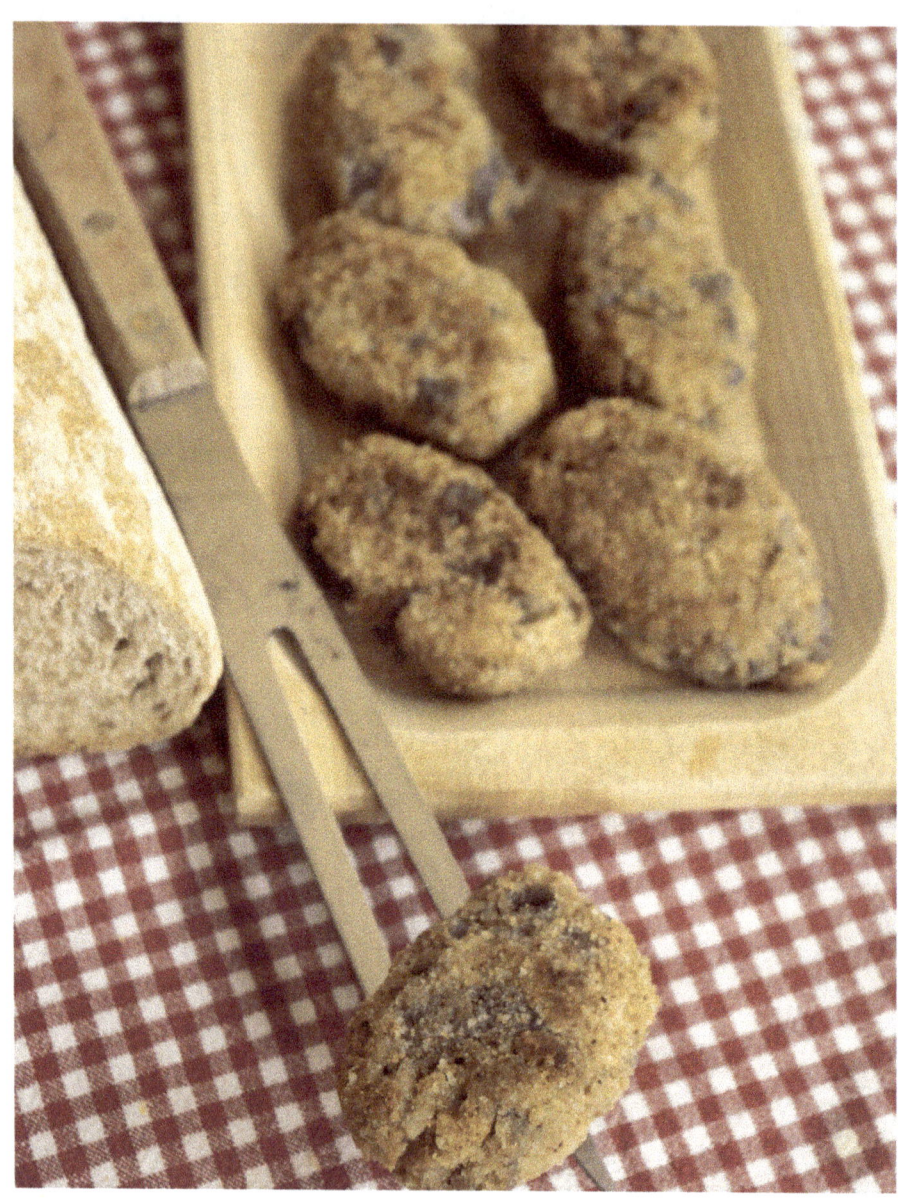

Spicy Artichoke

Prep Time: 10 min | **Cook Time:** 35 min | **Serve:** 2

- 2 artichokes, halved
- 1 teaspoon minced garlic
- ½ teaspoon ground coriander
- ¼ teaspoon dried thyme
- 1 teaspoon dried oregano
- 4 teaspoons olive oil

1. Put the artichokes in the tray.

2. Then rub them with minced garlic, ground coriander, dried thyme, and oregano.

3. Sprinkle the artichokes with olive oil and cook them at 350F for 35 minutes.

Nutrition: 161 calories, 5.5g protein, 18.1g carbohydrates, 9.7g fat, 9.2g fiber, 0mg cholesterol, 153mg sodium, 619mg potassium

Mushrooms Cakes

Prep Time: 10 min | **Cook Time:** 10 min | **Serve:** 8

- 3 cups mushrooms, sliced
- ½ cup almond flour
- 1 teaspoon chili flakes
- 1 teaspoon ground coriander
- 1 tablespoon olive oil
- ¼ cup plain yogurt

1. In the mixing bowl, mix sliced mushrooms with almond flour, chili flakes, ground coriander, and yogurt.
2. Then preheat the olive oil well in the skillet.
3. Make the small cakes from the mushroom mixture and put in the hot skillet.
4. Roast the mushroom cakes for 4 minutes per side.

Nutrition: 68 calories, 2.8g protein, 2.9g carbohydrates, 5.3g fat, 1g fiber, 0mg cholesterol, 9mg sodium, 102mg potassium

Baked Grapes

Prep Time: 10 min | **Cook Time:** 20 min | **Serve:** 6

- 3 cups green grapes
- 1 oz raisins, chopped
- 1 tablespoon olive oil
- 1 tablespoon lemon juice
- 1 teaspoon dried oregano

1. Mix grapes with raisins, olive oil, lemon juice, and dried oregano.

2. Put the mixture in the tray and bake at 360F for 20 minutes.

Nutrition: 66 calories, 0.5g protein, 11.8g carbohydrates, 2.6g fat, 0.7g fiber, 0mg cholesterol, 2mg sodium, 131mg potassium

Green Peas Paste

Prep Time: 10 min | **Cook Time:** 0 min | **Serve:** 4

- 2 cups green peas, boiled
- 1 tablespoon almond butter
- ¼ cup fresh parsley, chopped
- 2 tablespoons lemon juice

1. Put all ingredients in the blender and blend until smooth.
2. Transfer the mixture into the serving bowl.

Nutrition: 86 calories, 5g protein, 11.6g carbohydrates, 2.6g fat, 4.3g fiber, 0mg cholesterol, 8mg sodium, 237mg potassium

Baked Butternut Squash

Prep Time: 10 min | **Cook Time:** 35 min | **Serve:** 4

- 1-pound butternut squash, chopped
- 1 teaspoon ground ginger
- 1 teaspoon ground paprika
- 1 tablespoon olive oil

1. In the mixing bowl mix butternut squash with ground ginger, paprika, and olive oil.
2. Put the butternut squash mixture in the tray, flatten it well and bake at 360F for 35 minutes.

Nutrition: 84 calories, 1.3g protein, 13.9g carbohydrates, 3.7g fat, 2.5g fiber, 0mg cholesterol, 5mg sodium, 418mg potassium

Cauliflower Balls

Prep Time: 10 min | **Cook Time:** 16 min | **Serve:** 4

- 2 cups cauliflower, shredded
- 3 oz tofu, shredded
- 3 tablespoons almond flour
- 2 tablespoons coconut cream
- 1 teaspoon curry powder
- 1 tablespoon olive oil

1. In the mixing bowl, mix shredded cauliflower with tofu, almond flour, coconut cream, and curry powder.

2. Make the balls from the mixture.

3. Then preheat the skillet well.

4. Add olive oil.

5. Then add cauliflower balls in the hot oil and roast them for 4 minutes per side or until the balls are light brown.

Nutrition: 108 calories, 4.1g protein, 4.9g carbohydrates, 8.8g fat, 2.3g fiber, 0mg cholesterol, 21mg sodium, 210mg potassium

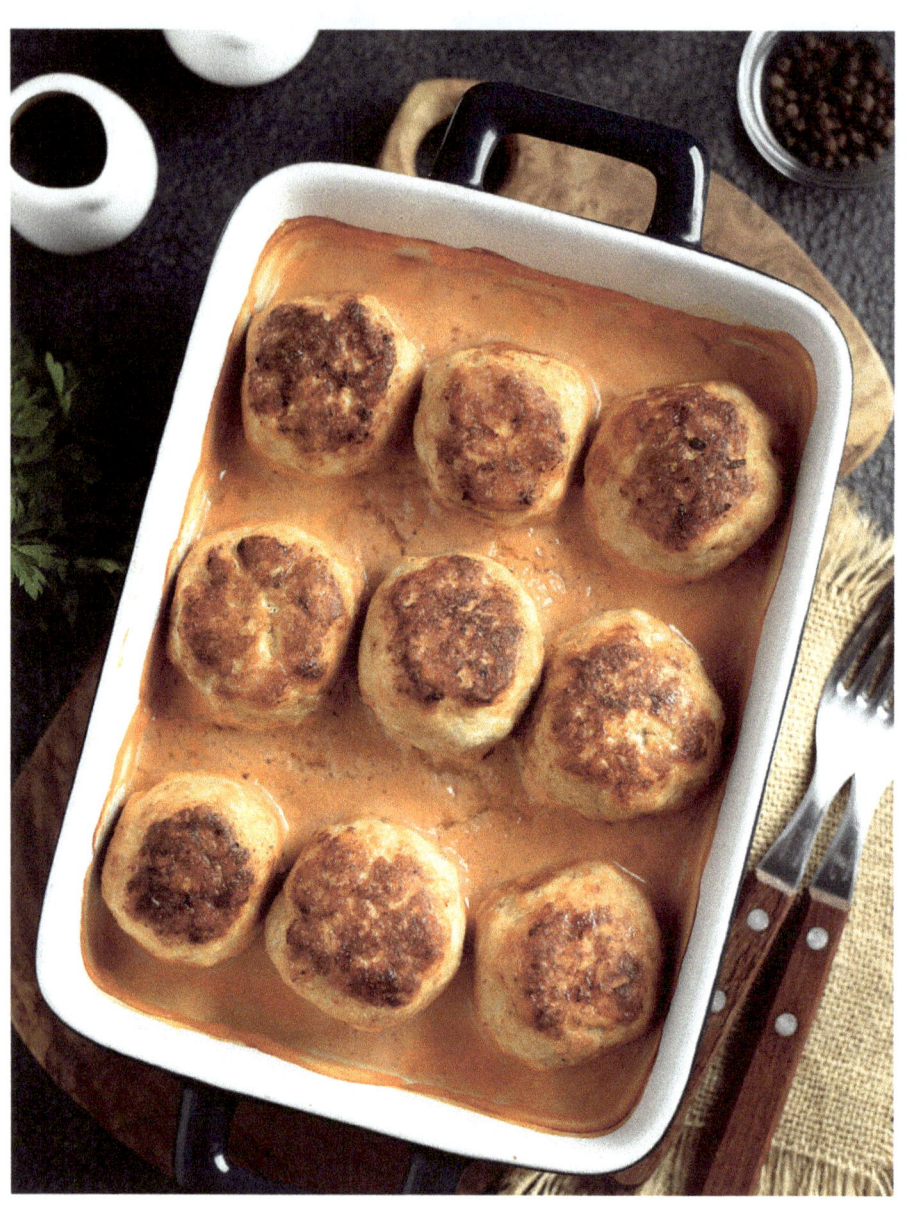

Baked Eggplants

Prep Time: 10 min | **Cook Time:** 30 min | **Serve:** 4

- 4 eggplants, halved
- 1 teaspoon minced garlic
- 2 tablespoons olive oil

1.Rub the eggplants with minced garlic and olive oil.

2.Put the eggplant halves in the tray and bake at 375F for 30 minutes.

Nutrition: 198 calories, 5.4g protein, 32.5g carbohydrates, 8g fat, 19.4g fiber, 0mg cholesterol, 11mg sodium, 1258mg potassium

Zucchini Cakes

Prep Time: 10 min | **Cook Time:** 15 min | **Serve:** 4

- 2 zucchinis, grated
- 3 tablespoons almond flour
- 1 teaspoon ground coriander
- 1 tablespoon olive oil

1. In the mixing bowl, mix grated zucchini with almond flour and ground coriander.
2. Preheat the skillet and pour the olive oil inside.
3. Preheat the oil.
4. Then make the cakes from the zucchini mixture and put them in the hot oil.
5. Cook the zucchini cakes for 3-4 minutes per side.

Nutrition: 77 calories, 2.3g protein, 4.4g carbohydrates, 6.2g fat, 1.6g fiber, 0mg cholesterol, 12mg sodium, 257mg potassium

Baked Jalapenos

Prep Time: 10 min | **Cook Time:** 20 min | **Serve:** 4

- 8 jalapenos, trimmed
- 1 tablespoon olive oil
- 1 teaspoon fennel seeds

1. Line the baking tray with baking paper.

2. Then put the jalapenos in the baking tray and sprinkle with olive oil and fennel seeds.

3. Bake the jalapenos at 375F for 20 minutes.

Nutrition: 40 calories, 0.5g protein, 1.9g carbohydrates, 3.7g fat, 1g fiber, 0mg cholesterol, 1mg sodium, 69mg potassium

Baked Onions

Prep Time: 10 min | **Cook Time:** 20 min | **Serve:** 4

- 4 red onions, peeled
- 1 teaspoon dried dill
- 1 teaspoon garlic powder
- 2 tablespoons olive oil

1. Make the cuts in the onions and sprinkle them with dried dill, garlic powder, and olive oil.
2. Then wrap the onions in the foil and put in the tray.
3. Bake the onions at 400F for 20 minutes.

Nutrition: 107 calories, 1.4g protein, 10.9g carbohydrates, 7.1g fat, 2.5g fiber, 0mg cholesterol, 5mg sodium, 177mg potassium

Mushroom Steaks

Prep Time: 10 min | **Cook Time:** 10 min | **Serve:** 2

- 2 Portobello mushrooms
- 1 tablespoon olive oil
- ½ teaspoon ground black pepper

1. Beat the mushrooms gently with the help of the kitchen hammer.

2. Then sprinkle the mushroom steaks with ground black pepper and olive oil.

3. Roast the mushrooms steaks in the well-preheat skillet for 5 minutes per side.

Nutrition: 81 calories, 3.1g protein, 3.3g carbohydrates, 7g fat, 1.1g fiber, 0mg cholesterol, 0mg sodium, 307mg potassium

Baked Turnip

Prep Time: 10 min | **Cook Time:** 35 min | **Serve:** 3

- 2 cups turnips, peeled, roughly chopped
- 1 tablespoon olive oil
- 1 teaspoon dried oregano

1. Put the turnip in the baking tray and flatten it gently.

2. Sprinkle the vegetables with olive oil and dried oregano.

3. Bake the turnip at 355F for 35 minutes.

Nutrition: 65 calories, 0.7g protein, 5.7g carbohydrates, 4.7g fat, 1.5g fiber, 0mg cholesterol, 53mg sodium, 162mg potassium

Avocado Spread

Prep Time: 10 min | **Cook Time:** 0 min | **Serve:** 2

- 1 avocado, pitted, chopped, peeled
- ¼ cup plain yogurt
- 1 garlic clove, diced

1. Put all ingredients in the blender and blend until smooth.
2. Transfer the spread in the serving bowl.

Nutrition: 229 calories, 3.8g protein, 11.3g carbohydrates, 20g fat, 6.8g fiber, 0mg cholesterol, 28mg sodium, 565mg potassium

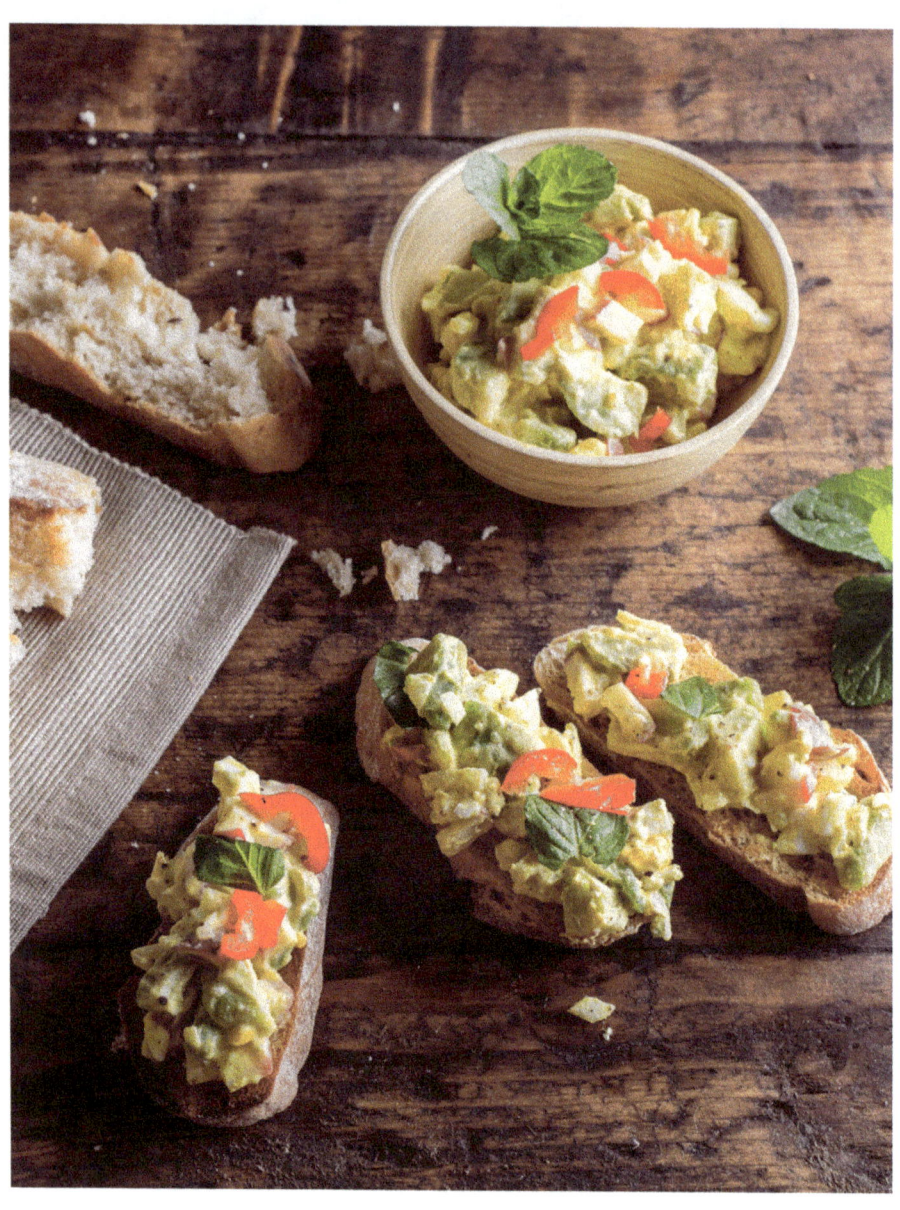

Burrito Bowl

Prep Time: 10 min | **Cook Time:** 0 min | **Serve:** 4

- 4 tomatoes, chopped
- 1 cucumber, chopped
- ¼ cup quinoa, cooked
- 2 tablespoons plain yogurt
- 1 teaspoon ground coriander
- 1 teaspoon chili powder
- ¼ cup fresh cilantro, chopped

1. Put all ingredients in the serving bowls and carefully mix them.

Nutrition: 81 calories, 3.7g protein, 15.4g carbohydrates, 1.2g fat, 2.9g fiber, 0mg cholesterol, 21mg sodium, 511mg potassium

Grilled Peppers

Prep Time: 10 min | **Cook Time:** 8 min | **Serve:** 4

- 4 sweet peppers
- 1 tablespoon olive oil
- 1 teaspoon fresh parsley, chopped
- 1 teaspoon sesame seeds

1. Preheat the grill to 400F.

2. Put the sweet peppers in the grill and cook for 4 minutes per side.

3. Then peel the sweet peppers and chop them roughly.

4. Mix the chopped peppers with olive oil, parsley, and sesame seeds.

Nutrition: 72 calories, 1.3g protein, 9.2g carbohydrates, 4.2g fat, 1.7g fiber, 0mg cholesterol, 3mg sodium, 229mg potassium

Parsley Guacamole

Prep Time: 10 min | **Cook Time:** 0 min | **Serve:** 4

- 1 avocado, pitted, peeled and chopped
- ½ cup chopped parsley
- 2 lemons
- ¼ cup coconut cream

1. Mix avocado with parsley and coconut cream.
2. Gently blend the mixture.
3. Then squeeze the lemon juice in the avocado mixture.
4. Carefully mix the meal.

Nutrition: 148 calories, 1.8g protein, 8.3g carbohydrates, 13.5g fat, 4.8g fiber, 0mg cholesterol, 10mg sodium, 365mg potassium

Baked Chickpeas

Prep Time: 10 min | **Cook Time:** 20 min | **Serve:** 4

- 2 cups chickpeas, boiled
- 1 tablespoon olive oil
- 1 teaspoon chili powder
- 1 teaspoon ground black pepper
- 1 tablespoon dried oregano

1. Line the baking tray with baking paper.
2. Then mix chickpeas with olive oil, chili powder, ground black pepper, and dried oregano.
3. Put the mixture in the baking tray and bake at 365F for 20 minutes.

Nutrition: 401 calories, 19.6g protein, 62.1g carbohydrates, 9.8g fat, 18.2g fiber, 0mg cholesterol, 31mg sodium, 913mg potassium

Broccoli Steaks

Prep Time: 10 min | **Cook Time:** 20 min | **Serve:** 4

- 1-pound broccoli head
- 1 teaspoon cayenne pepper
- 2 tablespoons olive oil

1. Slice the broccoli head into the steaks and put in the baking tray in one layer.
2. Sprinkle the vegetables with cayenne pepper and olive oil.
3. Bake the broccoli steaks at 365F for 10 minutes per side.

Nutrition: 100 calories, 3.2g protein, 7.8g carbohydrates, 7.5g fat, 3.1g fiber, 0mg cholesterol, 38mg sodium, 368mg potassium

Lemon Bok Choy

Prep Time: 10 min | **Cook Time:** 20 min | **Serve:** 4

- 1 pound bok choy, sliced
- 1 lemon
- 1 tablespoon olive oil
- 1 teaspoon cumin seeds

1. Preheat the olive oil in the skillet well.
2. Add bok choy and roast it for 1 minute per side.
3. Then sprinkle the bok choy with cumin seeds.
4. Squeeze the lemon juice over the bok choy, carefully mix the meal, and cook it on low heat for 15 minutes.

Nutrition: 51 calories, 2g protein, 4.1g carbohydrates, 3.9g fat, 1.6g fiber, 0mg cholesterol, 75mg sodium, 315mg potassium

Tomato & Mushroom Soup

Prep Time: 55 Minutes | **Serve:** 4-6

- 8Cups beef broth
- 1 Pound mushrooms (thin slices)
- 1 Garlic clove (minced)
- 6tbsp Butter
- 1 Can tomato sauce
- 2 Medium onions (chopped)
- 2 Medium tomatoes (peeled)
- 2 Chop carrots
- 2tbsp Salt & ½tbsp black pepper
- Sour cream
- 3tbsp fresh parsley
- 3 Celery ribs (chopped)

- 3tbsp All-purpose flour

1. Sautee mushrooms with butter in a large kettle on medium flame.

2. In the same pot, Sautee carrots, garlic, onion, and celery with butter.

3. Now add beef broth, half mushrooms, tomato sauce, and tomato slices. Simmer it almost for15 minutes on medium flame.

4. Now add parsley with remaining mushrooms and stir for 15 minutes. Mix all-purpose flour in water and add it gradually in it.

5. Simmer for 10 minutes. Garnish it with sour cream.

Broccoli & Cheese Soup

Prep Time: 40 Minutes | **Serve:** 4-5

- 1 Medium onion (chopped)
- ½ Cup butter
- 14ounces Chicken Broth
- 1 Loaf cheese food (processed)
- 1tbsp Garlic Powder
- 3 Cans frozen broccoli
- 2/3 Cup corn starch
- 2 Cups milk
- 1 Cup water

1.Melt butter in a pan on medium flame and cook the onion for 5 min.

2.In cooked onion add broccoli and chicken broth and stir for a few minutes.

3.Now add cheese cubes, garlic powder, and powder and cook it on low flame.

4.Mix cornstarch with water in a bowl and add it to the soup.

5.Simmer the soup for 15 minutes until all the cheese is melt.

6.Serve it hot with parsley and parmesan cheese

Red Lentils with Spinach

Prep Time: 15 min | **Cook Time:** 30 min | **Serve:** 4

- 3½ cups water
- 1½ cups red lentils, soaked for 20 minutes and drained
- ½ teaspoon red chili powder
- ½ teaspoon ground turmeric
- Salt, to taste
- 1-pound fresh spinach, chopped
- 2 tablespoons coconut oil
- 1 onion, chopped
- 1 teaspoon mustard seeds
- 1 teaspoon ground cumin
- ½ cup coconut milk
- 1 teaspoon garam masala

1. In a large pan, add water, lentils, red chili powder, turmeric and salt and bring to a boil on high heat.
2. Reduce the heat to low and simmer, covered for about 15 minutes.
3. Stir in spinach and simmer for about 5 minutes.
4. In a frying pan, melt coconut oil on medium heat.
5. Add onion, mustard seeds and cumin and sauté for about 4-5 minutes.
6. Transfer the onion mixture into the pan with the lentils and stir to combine.
7. Stir in coconut milk and garam masala and simmer for about 3-4 minutes.

Nutrition: Calories: 362, Fat: 14g, Sat Fat: 2g, Carbohydrates: 49g, Fiber: 13g, Sugar: 5g, Protein: 21g, Sodium: 693mg

Vegetarian Balls in Gravy

Prep Time: 20 min | **Cook Time:** 25 min | **Serve:** 4-6

For Balls:

- 1 cup cooked chickpeas
- 1 cup cooked red kidney beans
- ½ cup cooked quinoa
- Salt and freshly ground black pepper, to taste 2 tablespoons black beans flour 1 medium onion, chopped
- 2 garlic cloves, chopped
- ¼ cup fresh cilantro, chopped
- 1 teaspoon cumin seeds
- Pinch of baking soda
- 1 tablespoon fresh lemon juice

- 2 teaspoons olive oil

For Gravy:

- 1 teaspoon olive oil
- 1 teaspoon cumin seeds
- 1 medium onion, chopped finely
- 1 (1-inch) piece fresh ginger, grated finely
- 2 tomatoes, chopped finely
- 2 green chilies, chopped finely
- ½ teaspoon garam masala
- ½ teaspoon ground turmeric
- ½ teaspoon red chili powder
- Salt, to taste
- 2 cups water
- ¼ cup fresh cilantro, chopped

1. For balls in a food processor, add all ingredients except oil and pulse till a coarse meal forms.

2. Transfer the mixture into a bowl.

3. Cover the bowl with a foil paper and refrigerate for at least 1 hour.

4. Remove the mixture from refrigerator and make equal sized balls.

5. In a nonstick skillet, heat oil on medium heat.

6. Cook the balls for about 2-3 minutes or till golden brown from all sides.

7. For gravy in a nonstick pan, heat oil on medium heat.

8. Add cumin seeds and sauté for about 1 minute.

9. Add onion and sauté for about 6-7 minutes.

10. Stir in ginger, tomatoes, green chilies and spices and cook for about 1-2 minutes.

11. Add water and bring to a boil.

12. Reduce the heat to low and simmer, covered for about 10 minutes.

13. Carefully, place the balls in the gravy and cook for about 1-2 minutes.

14. Sprinkle with cilantro and serve.

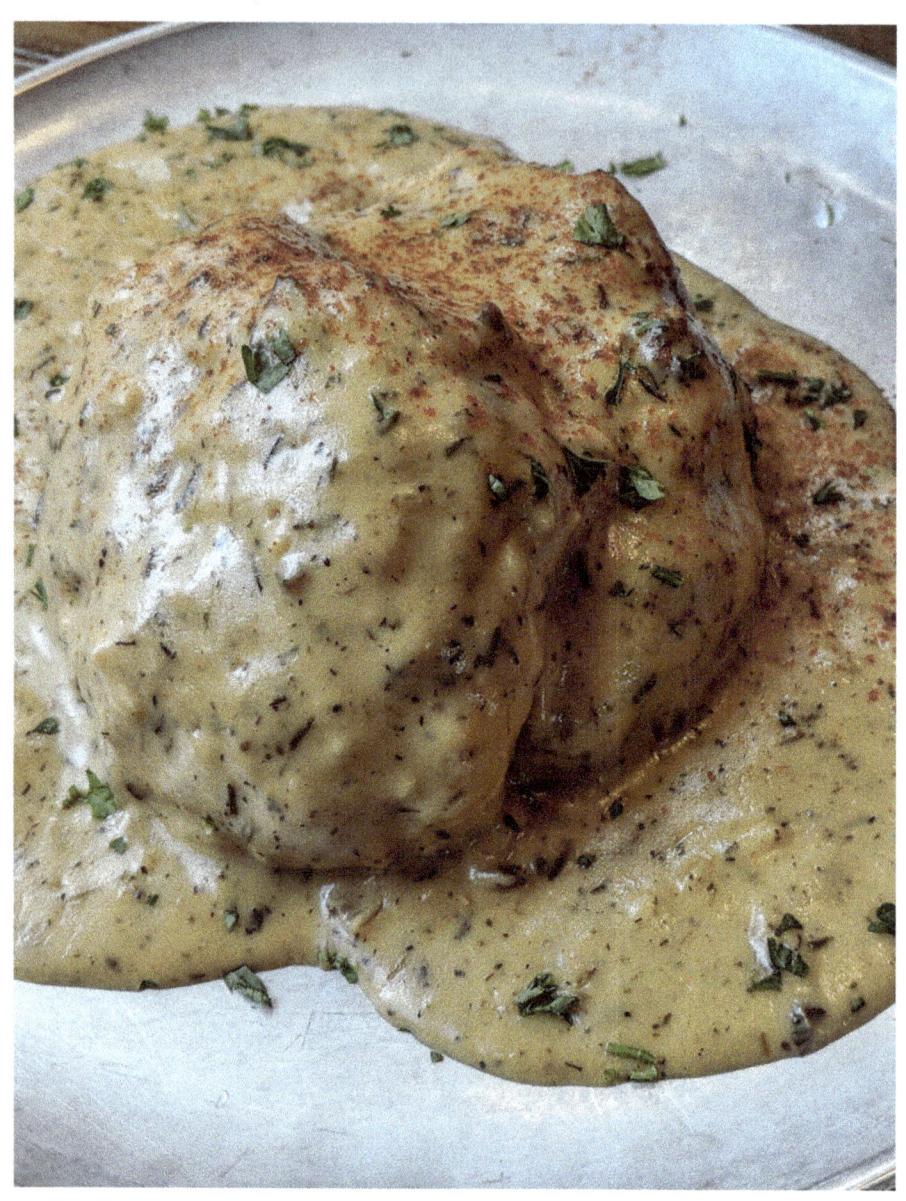

Quinoa with Veggies

Prep Time: 15 min | **Cook Time:** 35 min | **Serve:** 3

- 2 tablespoons olive oil
- 1 small onion, minced
- 2 carrots, peeled and sliced
- 1 celery stalk, chopped
- 1 garlic clove, minced
- ½ cup uncooked quinoa, rinsed
- 1 teaspoon ground turmeric
- ¼ teaspoon dried basil, crushed
- Salt, to taste
- 1 cup vegetable broth
- 1 teaspoon fresh lime juice

1. In a pan, heat oil on medium heat.

2. Add onion, carrot, celery and garlic and sauté for about t minutes.

3. Stir in remaining ingredients except lime juice and bring to a gentle simmer.

4. Reduce the heat to low and simmer, covered for about 25-30 minutes or till all the liquid is absorbed.

5. Stir in lime juice and serve.

Nutrition: Calories: 227, Fat: 11g, Sat Fat: 5g, Carbohydrates: 23g, Fiber: 32, Sugar: 2g, Protein: 2g, Sodium: 195mg

Quinoa with Asparagus

Prep Time: 15 min | **Cook Time:** 18 min | **Serve:** 4

- 1-pound fresh asparagus, trimmed
- 2 teaspoons coconut oil
- ½ of onion, chopped
- 2 minced garlic cloves
- 1 cup cooked red quinoa
- 1 tablespoon ground turmeric
- ½ cup reduced-sodium vegetable broth
- ½ cup nutritional yeast
- 1 tablespoon fresh lemon juice

1. In a large pan of boiling water, cook the asparagus for about 2-3 minutes.

2.Drain well and rinse under cold water.

3.In a large skillet, melt coconut oil on medium heat.

4.Add onion and garlic and sauté for about 5 minutes.

5.Stir in quinoa, turmeric and broth and cook for about 5-6 minutes.

6.Stir in nutritional yeast, lemon juice and asparagus and cook for about 3-4 minutes.

Nutrition: Calories: 166, Fat: 2g, Sat Fat: 1g, Carbohydrates: 21g, Fiber: 9g, Sugar: 9g, Protein: 13g, Sodium: 37mg

Quinoa & Beans with Veggies

Prep Time: 20 min | **Cook Time:** 26 min | **Serve:** 6

- 2 cups water
- 1 cup dry quinoa
- 2 tablespoons coconut oil
- 1 medium onion, chopped
- 4 garlic cloves, chopped finely
- 2 tablespoons curry powder
- ½ teaspoon ground turmeric
- Cayenne pepper, to taste
- Salt, to taste
- 2 cups broccoli, chopped
- 1 cup fresh kale, trimmed and chopped
- 1 cup green peas, shelled

- 1 red bell pepper, seeded and chopped
- 2 cups canned kidney beans, rinsed and drained
- 2 tablespoons fresh lime juice

1. In a pan, add water and bring to a boil on high heat.
2. Add quinoa and reduce the heat to low.
3. Simmer for about 10-15 minutes or till all the liquid is absorbed.
4. In a large skillet, melt coconut oil on medium heart.
5. Add onion, garlic, curry powder, turmeric, salt, and sauté for about 4-5 minutes.
6. Add the vegetables and cook for about 5-6 minutes.
7. Stir in quinoa and beans,
8. Drizzle with lime juice and serve.

Coconut Brown Rice

Prep Time: 15 min | **Cook Time:** 1 hour | **Serve:** 14

- 12 cups water
- 1 tablespoon dried turmeric
- 2 pound brown rice
- 2 (13½-ounce) cans lite coconut milk
- 2 (13½-ounce) cans coconut milk
- 1 tablespoon fresh ginger, minced
- 1½ teaspoons fresh lemon zest, grated finely 4 dried bay leaves
- Salt and freshly ground black pepper, to taste Chopped cashews, for garnishing
- Chopped fresh cilantro, for garnishing

1. In a small bowl, add water and turmeric and beat till well combined.

2. In a large pan, add turmeric water and remaining ingredients except cashews and stir well.

3. Bring to a boil on high heat.

4. Reduce the heat to medium and simmer, stirring occasionally for about 30-35 minutes.

5. Reduce the heat to low and simmer, covered for about 20-25 minutes.

6. Remove bay leaf before serving.

7. Garnish with cashews and cilantro and serve.

Nutrition: Calories: 184, Fat: 2g, Carbohydrates: 27g, Fiber: 7g, Sugar: 9g, Protein: 2g, Sodium: 76mg,

Brown Rice & Cherries Pilaf

Prep Time: 20 min | **Cook Time:** 35 min | **Serve:** 8

- 1 (14-ounce) can low-sodium vegetable broth 1/3 cup water
- 1 cup brown basmati rice
- 1 tablespoon curry powder
- ½ teaspoon ground turmeric
- Pinch of saffron threads, crumbled
- 1/3 cup fresh lemon juice
- 3 tablespoons olive oil
- 3 tablespoons raw honey
- 1 tablespoon fresh ginger, minced
- 1 tablespoon fresh orange zest, grated finely Salt, to taste

- ¾ cup celery stalk, chopped
- ½ cup scallion, chopped, divided
- ¾ cup dried cherries, chopped roughly
- 1 cup fresh dark sweet cherries, pitted and chopped
- ¾ cup unsalted mixed nuts

1. In a pan, mix broth, water, rice, curry powder, turmeric and saffron and bring to a boil on medium-high heat.
2. Reduce the heat to low and simmer, covered for about 35 minutes.
3. Remove from heat and keep aside, covered for about 5 minutes.
4. With a fork, fluff the rice.
5. In a large glass bowl, mix lemon juice, oil, honey, ginger, orange zest and salt.
6. Stir in cooked rice, celery, ¼ cup of scallion and dried cherries.

7.Serve immediately with the topping of fresh cherries, nuts and remaining scallion.

Nutrition: Calories: 288, Fat: 12g, Sat Fat: 1g, Carbohydrates: 41g, Fiber: 5g, Protein: 6g, Sodium: 125mg

Brown Rice Casserole

Prep Time: 15 min | **Cook Time:** 1 hour | **Serve:** 2

- 1 teaspoon extra-virgin olive oil
- 1 red onion, sliced thinly
- 1½ teaspoons ground turmeric
- 9-ounce brown mushrooms, sliced
- 1 teaspoon raisins
- ½ cup brown rice, rinsed
- 1¼ cups vegetable broth
- ¼ cup fresh cilantro, chopped
- ½ tablespoons pine nuts, toasted
- 1 tablespoon fresh lemon juice
- Salt and freshly ground black pepper, to taste

Preheat the oven to 400 degrees F.

1. In an ovenproof casserole, heat oil on medium heat.

2. Add onion and turmeric and sauté for about 3 minutes.

3. Add mushrooms and stir fry for about 2 minutes.

4. Stir in raisins, rice and broth and transfer into oven.

5. Bake for about 45-55 minutes or till desired doneness.

6. Just before serving, stir in remaining ingredients.

Nutrition: Calories: 201, Fat: 5g, Sat Fat: 6g, Carbohydrates: 37g, Fiber: 5g, Sugar: 18g, Protein: 7g, Sodium: 384mg

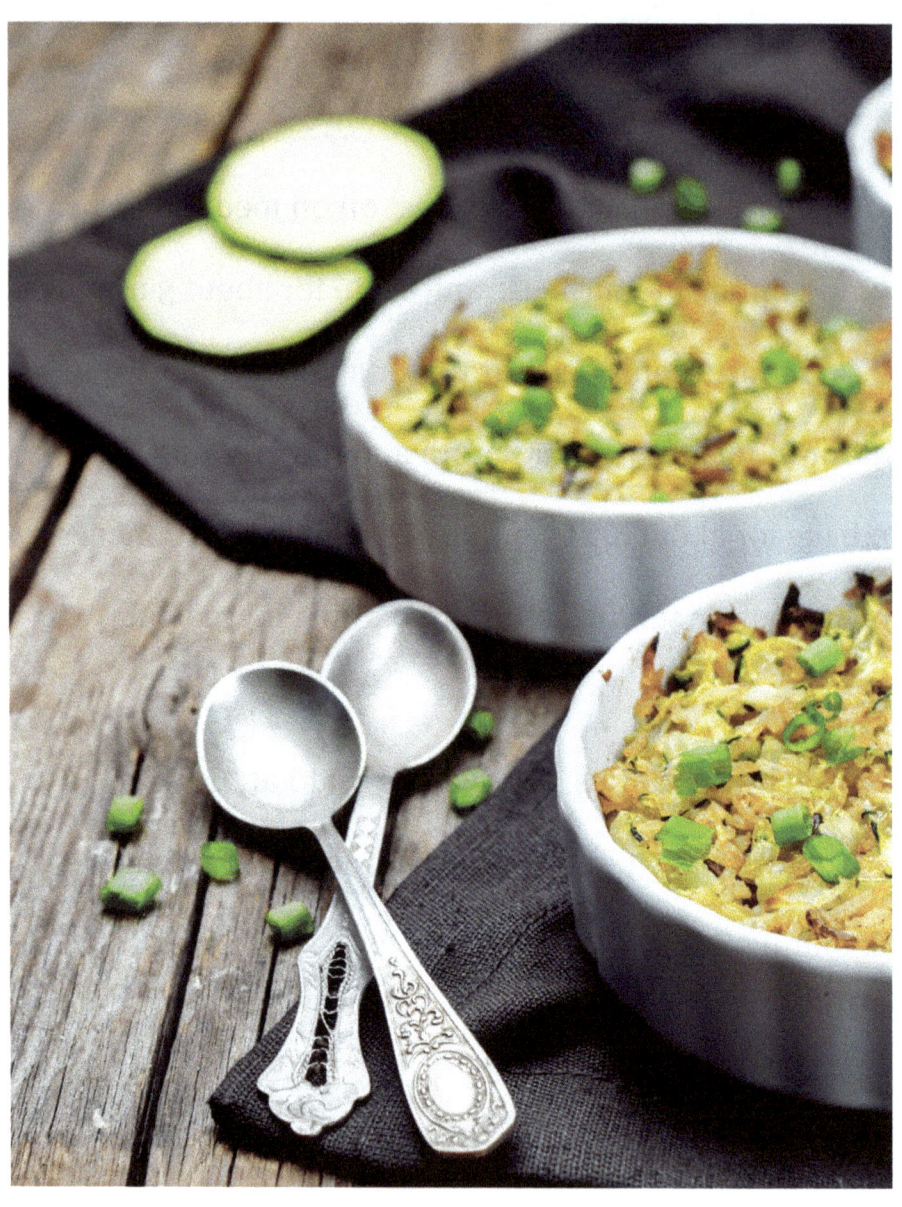

Rice, Lentils & Veggie Casserole

Prep Time: 20 min | **Cook Time:** 1 h 36 m | **Serve:** 10

- 3¾ cups water, divided
- ½ cup brown lentils, rinsed
- ½ cup wild rice, rinsed
- 1 tbsp olive oil
- ½ of medium onion, chopped
- 1 cup button mushrooms, sliced
- 1 cup tomato sauce
- 1 (10-ounce) package frozen spinach, thawed and squeezed
- 1 (16-ounce) package frozen peas, thawed
- 2 minced garlic cloves

- 1 tablespoon dried oregano, crushed
- 1 teaspoon smoked paprika
- ½ teaspoon ground turmeric
- ¼ cup nutritional yeast

For Sauce

- 1¼ cups unsweetened almond milk
- 1 cup unsalted cashews, soaked for 30 minutes and drained
- 1 teaspoon coconut aminos
- ½ teaspoon dried garlic

1. In a pan, add 3 ½ cups of water, lentils and rice and bring to a boil.

2. Reduce the heat to low and simmer, covered for about 35 minutes.

3. Remove from heat and keep aside to cool.

4. Preheat the oven to 350 degrees F. Grease a 13x9-inch casserole dish.

5. In a large skillet, heat 2 tablespoons of water on high heat.

6. Add onion and sauté for about 2-3 minutes.

7. Add mushrooms and cook for about 2 minutes.

8. Add remaining 2 tablespoons of water and remaining ingredients except nutritional yeast and cook for about 1 minute.

9. Remove from heat and mix with rice mixture.

10. Transfer the mixture into prepared casserole dish evenly.

11. In a blender, add all sauce ingredients and pulse till smooth.

12. Spread the sauce over the rice mixture evenly and stir to combine well.

13. Top with nutritional yeast evenly.

14. Bake for about 45 minutes.

Herbed Bulgur Pilaf

Prep Time: 20 min | **Cook Time:** 35 min | **Serve:** 6

- 2 tablespoons extra-virgin olive oil
- 2 cups onion, chopped
- 1 garlic clove, minced
- 1½ cups medium bulgur
- ½ teaspoon ground cumin
- ½ teaspoon ground turmeric
- 1½ cups carrot, peeled and chopped
- 2 teaspoons fresh ginger, grated finely
- Salt, to taste
- 2 cups vegetable broth
- 3 tablespoons fresh lemon juice
- ¼ cup fresh parsley, chopped

- ¼ cup fresh mint leaves, chopped
- ¼ cup fresh dill, chopped
- ½ cup walnuts, toasted and chopped

1. In a large deep skillet, heat oil on medium-low heat.
2. Add onion and cook, stirring occasionally for about 12-18 minutes.
3. Add garlic and sauté fir about 1 minute.
4. Add bulgur, cumin and turmeric and stir fry for about 1 minute.
5. Add carrot, ginger, salt and broth and bring to a boil, stirring occasionally.
6. Simmer, covered for about 15 minutes.
7. Remove from heat and keep aside, covered for about 5 minutes.

8.Stir in lemon juice and fresh herbs and serve with the garnishing of walnuts.

Nutrition: Calories: 277, Fat: 12g, Sat Fat: 1g, Carbohydrates: 39g, Fiber: 10g, Protein: 7g, Sodium: 507mg

Zoodles

Prep Time: 5 min | **Cook Time:** 0 min | **Serve:** 2

- Zucchini 4 organic

Directions- Zoodle Creation

1. If you have access to a spiralizer, use it to create noodles of zucchini. If you do not own a spiralizer, this recipe is still very simple. Just slice the zucchini into long thin strips. You may also wish to use a cheese and vegetable grater to get the desired noodle effect.
2. Serve the zoodles as they are or let them boil for two minutes in a pan of water to warm them up and soften them a bit. Alternately, you may wish to sauté them in a bit of coconut oil or Coconut oil for a minute or two to

give them a little crispness.

3.Serve the zoodles in place of the traditional noodles in your favorite pasta dishes.

Biryani

Prep Time: 15 min | **Cook Time:** 15 min | **Serve:** 6

- Black pepper as desired
- Sea salt as desired
- Garam masala .5 tsp
- Coconut oil 1 tsp
- Shelled peas 1 c
- Water 5 c
- Coriander .5 tsp ground
- Chili powder 1 tsp
- Turmeric 5 tsp
- Carrots 2 quartered
- Potatoes 2 quartered
- Bay leaves 2 torn

- Cumin seeds .5 tsp
- Onion 1 sliced thin
- Vegetable oil 3 T
- White rice long grain 2 c

1. Add the rice to a large pot and cover it with three to four inches of water before allowing it to soak for about 20 minutes. Drain and set aside.

2. Add the oil to your pressure cooker and set it over medium heat. Add in the onion, bay leaves, and cumin seeds and let everything cook about 5 minutes until the onion is nearly see through.

3. Mix in the carrots and potatoes and cook an additional 5 minutes and the potatoes have begun to brown. Add in the coriander, turmeric and chili powder and let everything cook 1 additional minute.

4. Add the rice to the pressure cooker and ensure it is well

covered in the boil before adding peas and water. Mix in the garam masala, oil, and salt before sealing the cooker and turning it to high pressure. Let everything cook for 5 minutes before removing from heat.

5. Allow the pressure to naturally release and fluff the rice with a fork before serving.

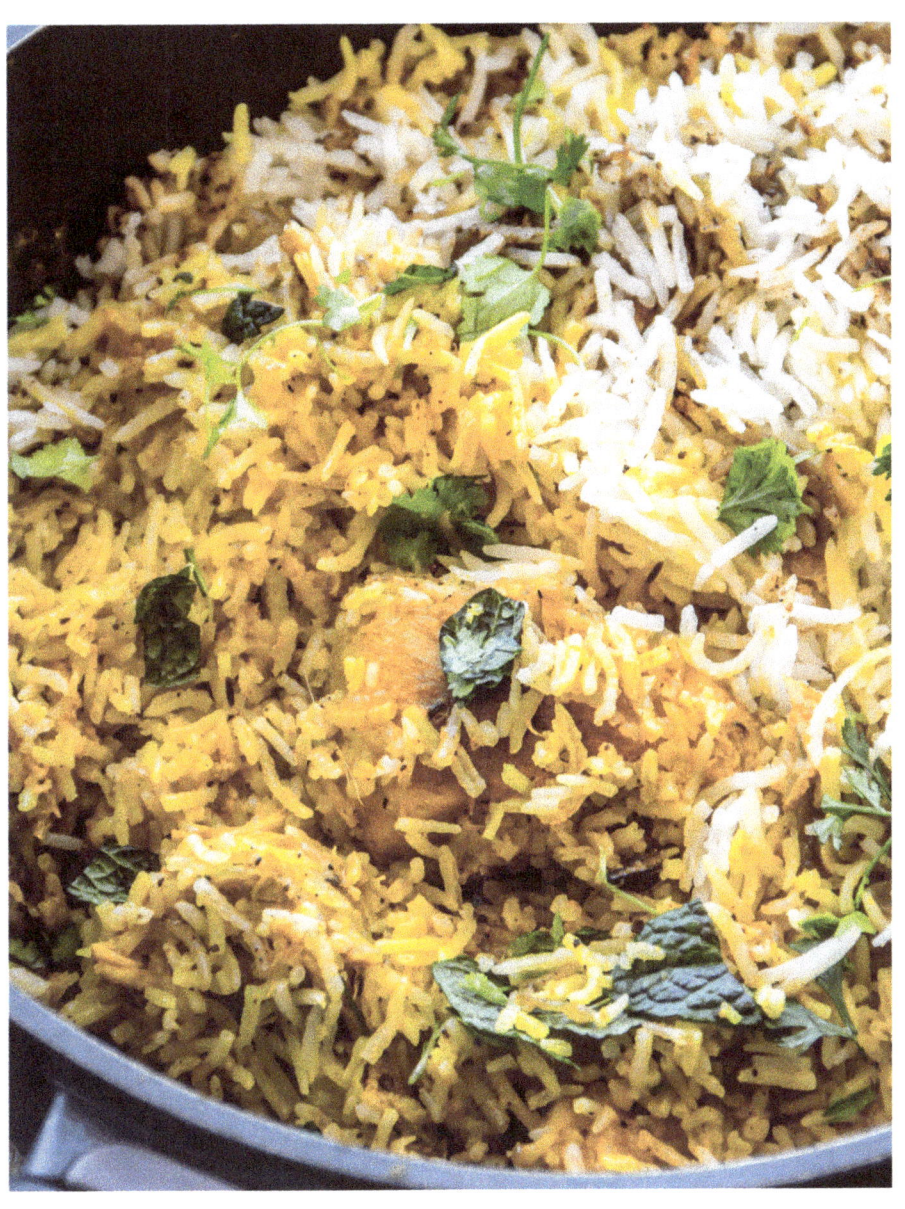

Greek Mixed Roasted Vegetables

Prep Time: 15 min | **Cook Time:** 45 min | **Serve:** 4

Ingredients- Vegetables

- 1 eggplant peeled and diced .75-inch
- Black pepper as desired
- Kosher sea salt as desired
- Extra virgin olive oil 2 T
- Garlic 2 cloves minced
- Onion 1 peeled, diced 1-inch
- Bell pepper 2 red, yellow, diced, 1-inch

Ingredients- Dressing

- Coconut oil .25 c
- Lemon juice .3 c squeezed fresh
- Black pepper as desired
- Kosher sea salt as desired
- Basil 15 leaves
- Scallions 4 minced

1.Ensure your oven is heated to 425F.

2.One a sheet pan, combine the garlic, onion, yellow bell pepper, red bell pepper, and eggplant before seasoning using the pepper, salt, and coconut oil.

3.Add the pan to the oven and let it cook for 40 minutes, using a spatula to flip everything after 20 minutes.

4. As the vegetables are cooking, combine the pepper, salt, coconut oil, and lemon juice in a small bowl and add the vegetables' results as soon as they are ready.

5. Let the pan cool completely before adding in the basil, feta, and scallions. Season before serving.

Autumn Roasted Green Beans

Prep Time: 15 min | **Cook Time:** 30 min | **Serve:** 4

- Walnuts .5 c toasted
- Cranberries .5 c dried
- Black pepper as desired
- Kosher sea salt as desired
- Lemon juice 2 tsp.
- Lemon zest 1 tsp.
- Sugar .25 tsp.
- Coconut oil 2 T
- Garlic 4 cloves, quartered and peeled
- Green beans 2 lbs. stems trimmed

1. Preheat your oven to 350F and crack and smash the walnuts into chunks.

2. Spread the walnuts onto a baking sheet and toast them for 10 minutes.

3. Increase the temperature on the oven to 450F.

4. Cover a baking sheet with a rim using aluminum foil.

5. In a mixing bowl, combine the sugar, pepper, salt, and coconut oil before thoroughly coating the garlic and green beans.

6. Place the beans onto a baking sheet and spread them out to ensure they cook well. Place the sheet into the oven and let the beans bake for 15 minutes, before stirring with a spatula and roasting another 10 minutes.

7. Mix in the lemon juice, pepper and salt before serving.

Roasted Summer Squash

Prep Time: 5 min | **Cook Time:** 30 min | **Serve:** 4

- Zucchini 3
- Yellow squash 3
- Kosher salt 5 T
- Black pepper .5 T
- Coconut oil 2 T

1. Ensure your oven is heated to 400F

2. Peel vegetables and cut into .25 inch thick slices.

3. Assemble vegetables on a baking sheet or pan and drizzle coconut oil on top. Sprinkle with seasoning as desired

4. Bake at 400F for 30 minutes.

Savory Baked Acorn Squash

Prep Time: 5 min | **Cook Time:** 30 min | **Serve:** 4

- Acorn squash 1
- Kosher salt as desired
- Black pepper as desired
- Coconut oil 2 tsp.
- Smoked paprika as desired

1. Ensure your oven is heated to 425F.
2. Cut acorn squash in half lengthwise, then cut halves into quarters lengthwise. Scoop out seeds and discard.
3. Place the squash on baking sheet and drizzle coconut oil over the top of each quarter. Scatter with the smoked paprika, salt, and pepper and bake in the oven for 30 minutes.

Roasted Brussels Sprouts

Prep Time: 5 min | **Cook Time:** 15 min | **Serve:** 4

- Sea salt .25 tsp.
- Black pepper .25 tsp.
- Brussel sprouts .75lbs. sliced in half length-wise
- Coconut oil 5 T.

1.Ensure your oven is heated to 400F. Cut Brussels sprouts in half and place in a medium-sized bowl. Drizzle the coconut oil over the Brussels sprouts and then toss with the sea salt and black pepper until evenly coated.

2.Pour Brussels sprouts onto a baking sheet and make sure they are evenly spaced so that they will roast easily.

3.Place the sheet in the oven and let it cook

approximately 10 minutes before stirring well and returning it to the oven for 10 minutes more. Season as desired They will keep in the fridge for 3-4 days, or in the freezer for 2-3 months.

Roasted Rosemary Potatoes

Prep Time: 10 min | **Cook Time:** 25 min | **Serve:** 6

- Garlic 1 head
- Rosemary 3 sprigs
- Thyme 3 sprigs
- Baby potatoes 20 oz.
- Parsley 2 T chopped
- Sea salt as desired
- Black pepper as desired
- Coconut oil 2 T

1.Ensure your oven is heated to 450F.

2.Separate garlic cloves and remove the papery skin holding them together, but do not peel.

3. Add the rosemary, thyme, baby potatoes, parsley, garlic, and coconut oil together in a large bowl, coating well.

4. Add the results to a jelly roll pan that has been lined with tinfoil before topping with pepper and salt. Place the pan in the oven and let the potatoes bake approximately 25 minutes, stirring at the 12-minute mark.

5. Season with additional pepper and salt before serving.

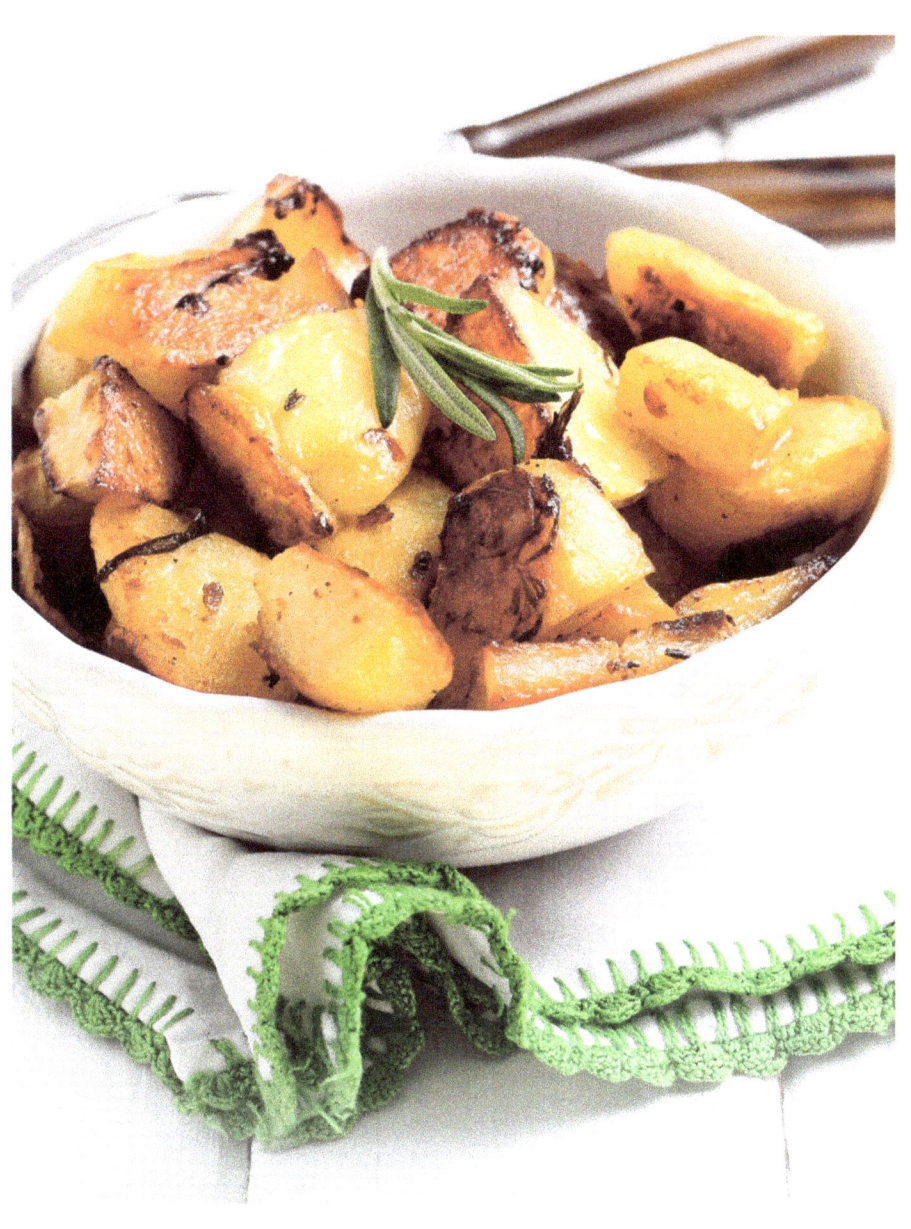

Sweet Potato Wedges

Prep Time: 10 min | **Cook Time:** 30 min | **Serve:** 6

- Salt 1 tsp.
- Cracked black pepper 1 tsp.
- Garlic powder .5 tsp.
- Sweet potatoes 4 medium, peeled, each cut into 6 wedges
- Rosemary 1 T chopped, fresh
- Coconut oil 2 T

1. Preheat oven to 450F.

2. In a mixing bowl, combine the coconut oil, rosemary, sweet potatoes, garlic powder, black pepper, and salt and ensure the potatoes are coated well.

3.Add the results in a single layer to a large roasting pan before placing the pan in the oven and letting the potatoes bake for 20 minutes. Turn the dish at this point before baking another 10 minutes.

Best Lentil Curry

Prep Time: 10 min | **Cook Time:** 30 min | **Serve:** 4

- Vegetable broth 4 c low sodium
- Red lentil 1 c
- Potato 10 oz. peeled and made into pieces that are 1 inch each
- Carrot 8 oz. chopped
- Curry powder 1 T
- Scallions 8 separated, sliced
- Garlic 2 cloves chopped
- Ginger 2 T chopped
- Coconut oil 3 T

1. Add the oil to a saucepan before placing it on the stove on top of a burner set to a high/medium heat.

2.Add in the scallion whites, garlic and ginger and let them soften for 2 minutes.

3.Mix in the curry powder and pepper and salt, as desired, broth, lentils, potato, and carrots before letting everything boil. Turn down the heat and let everything simmer for 15 minutes, stirring regularly.

4.Top with scallion greens before serving.

Chana Masala

Prep Time: 5 min | **Cook Time:** 25 min | **Serve:** 4

- Curry powder 1 tsp.
- Chickpeas 32 oz. rinsed, drained
- Garlic 2 cloves minced
- Onion 1 large, chopped
- Extra virgin olive oil 1 T
- Cilantro .25 c
- Kosher sea salt as desired
- Lemon juice 1 T
- Tomatoes 2 chopped
- Ginger 2 tsp. grated
- Turmeric .5 tsp.

1. Add the oil to a skillet before placing it on a burner set to a medium/high heat. Add in the onion and let it sauté until it has become translucent and soft. Mix in the garlic and let it cook for 3 minutes.

2. Add in the curry powder, chickpeas, coconut oil, lemon juice, tomatoes, ginger and turmeric along with .25 c of water. Let the mixture simmer before cooking it for 10 minutes, stirring on occasion. The result should have a stew-like consistency but not be runny.

3. Season using salt and top with cilantro before serving.

Zucchini Noodle Pasta with Avocado Pesto

Prep Time: 30 min | **Cook Time:** 15 min | **Serve:** 8

- Zucchinis 6 spiralized
- Cold pressed oil of choice 1 T

Ingredients- Pesto

- Pine nuts .25 c
- Avocados 2 cubed
- Parsley .25 c leaves
- Basil 1 c leaves
- Garlic 3 cloves
- Lemon juice 1 lemon
- Cold pressed oil of choice 3 T

- Salt as desired
- Pepper as desired

1. Spiralize your zucchini and set aside on paper towels.
2. In a food processor, add in all ingredients for the avocado pesto except the oil. Pulse on low until desired consistency is reached.
3. Slowly add in coconut oil until creamy and emulsified.
4. Heat 1 T and your zucchini noodles cook for 4 min.
5. Take your zucchini noodles and coat with avocado pesto.

Thai Soup

Prep Time: 30 min | **Cook Time:** 15 min | **Serve:** 9

- Spiralized Zucchinis 2 medium
- Minced Garlic Cloves 2 total
- Thin Sliced Red Pepper 1 total
- Diced Jalapeno 1 total
- Lime 1 cut into 8 wedges
- Thin Sliced Onion 5 total
- Full-Fat Coconut Milk 15oz
- Vegetable Broth 6 c
- Fresh Chopped Cilantro 5 c
- Green Curry Paste 5 T
- Coconut Oil 1 T

1. Add the coconut oil to a saucepan before adding in the onions and letting them sauté. Takes about 5 minutes.

2. Add jalapeno, curry paste, and minced garlic. Sauté for 1 minute or until just fragrant. Stir in bone broth and coconut milk, mix until thoroughly combined. Heat until soup comes to a boil and then reduce to medium heat. Add red pepper slices, then mix.

3. Simmer soup approximately 5 minutes or until done, until chicken is cooked through. Add fresh cilantro.

4. Divide zucchini into 8 bowls and ladle soup over them. The heat of the soup will cook the zucchini noodles. If not serving all at once, store soup and zoodles separately and combine when prepared to eat, so zoodles don't become soggy.

Vegan Lasagna

Prep Time: 10 min | **Cook Time:** 4 hours | **Serve:** 8

- Lasagna Zoodles 6
- Vegan cheese 5 c
- Red pepper flakes .25 tsp.
- Basil .5 tsp. dried
- Oregano 1 tsp. dried
- Salt 1 tsp.
- Tomato sauce 15 oz.
- Tomato 28 oz. crushed
- Garlic 1 clove minced
- Onion 1 chopped
- Ground soy 1 lb.

1.Place a skillet on the stove on top of a burner set to a high/medium heat before adding garlic, onion, and soy and letting the soy brown.

2.Add in the red pepper flakes, basil, oregano, salt, tomato sauce, and crushed tomatoes and let the results simmer 5 minutes.

3.Add.3 of the total sauce from the skillet and add it to the slow cooker. Place 3 Zoodles on top of the sauce, followed by cheese mixture. Create three layers in total.

4.Cover the slow cooker and let it cook on a low heat for 6 hours.

Caprese Zoodles

Prep Time: 10 min | **Cook Time:** 15 min | **Serve:** 4

- Zucchini 4 large
- 2 T coconut oil
- Kosher salt as desired
- Black pepper as desired
- Cherry tomatoes, 2 c halved
- Mozzarella balls 1 c quartered
- Basil leaves .25 c torn
- Balsamic vinegar 2 T

1. Place the zoodles in a serving bowl before adding in the coconut oil and tossing well. Season as desired and allow the zoodles to marinate for at least 15 minutes.

2.Mix in the basil, mozzarella, and tomatoes and toss well.

3.Top with balsamic before serving.

www.ingramcontent.com/pod-product-compliance
Lightning Source LLC
Chambersburg PA
CBHW070733030426
42336CB00013B/1960